Smart Points Cookbook

50 Smart Points Weight Watchers Recipes

Dinner Meals Low on Points But Packed with Flavor

By: Robert Edeson

Table Of Contents

Introduction

Are you constantly searching for a more effective weight loss plan that will help you get fit without starving? Or have you always wanted to learn how to cook healthy dinners that will positively change your life? If your answer to any of these questions is yes, then this book is just for you as it contains 50 SmartPoints recipes that are low in points but high on flavor and nourishment. These recipes were inspired by the SmartPoints program of Weight Watchers which promotes cleaner eating, regular exercise and having a support system for successful weight loss.

The last quarter of 2015 unearthed a new and more credible system of counting food points which Weight Watchers called the SmartPoints. Compared to the former PointsPlus system, SmartPoints uses a new set of nutrients in calculating the point value of each food item. Instead of focusing on broad categories such as carbohydrates and fats, the new system is more specific as it uses calories, sugar, saturated fat and protein to measure and establish the nutritional weight-loss value of every meal that we eat.

The SmartPoints program is perfect for those who want to experience long-term weight loss without having to skip meals or count calories. It simply guides people to eat within their personal points allowance but nudges them to choose healthier and more organic ingredients such as fruits, vegetables, eggs, healthy oils and lean protein. These low SmartPoints ingredients contain powerful nutrients that trigger weight loss and better health.

The initial chapters of this book will show you essential information about the SmartPoints system including its features, benefits and method of computing food points. You will likewise be given a brief background on how a simple housewife named Jean Nidetch started the Weight Watchers empire in her own home in Queens, New York.

Moreover, this book contains 50 dinner recipes that are low in SmartPoints, thus making it healthier, lower in calories and tastier than unhealthy, fattening dishes. These recipes include salads, soups, poultry, beef, pork and seafood. Each recipe has a corresponding SmartPoints value for your own convenience. Once you try cooking these dishes, you will realize that there can be a healthy balance between weight loss and food, and that is the new SmartPoints system.

Thanks again for buying this book, I hope you enjoy it!

Chapter 1 Smart Points: The Key to Losing Weight and Loving Food

"I don't feel like I'm on a diet that I'm ever going to go off again;
I feel like I'll be counting points for the rest of my life."

Oprah Winfrey
Media mogul, philanthropist and
Weight Watchers spokesperson

2015 was a big year for American weight loss company Weight Watchers as it revamped its successful PointsPlus system into a more plausible method of counting food points, which they called the SmartPoints system. This latest method still promotes Weight Watcher's philosophy of helping people lose weight by teaching them to eat right, exercise more and build a support system with its other members.

However, what makes SmartPoints different from PointsPlus is that it shifted its focus on nutrients that have a direct impact on a person's fitness. In turn, people who choose to undergo this program are pressed to eat cleaner, leaner and more organic which will eventually have long-term benefits on one's health.

Before we delve into the new SmartPoints system, let us briefly revisit the humble beginnings of this multi-million dollar weight loss company.

Weight Watcher Beginnings

In 1961, an overweight stay-at-home mom by the name of Jean Nidetch regularly gathered a few of her closest friends in her house in Queens, New York. They communed over food obsessions and their experiences with fad diets. These friendly gatherings snowballed into larger support groups because more people wanted to join their discussions. More importantly, attendees of these meetings, including Jean herself, started to lose weight due to the mutual support and sharing of ideas that occurred.

This simple yet empathic way of coping with weight issues became the foundation of the Weight Watchers Company that officially started in 1963. This once humble American organization is now a multi-million dollar company which boasts of having more than one million members in over 30 countries. Its meal plans, nutritional point systems, recipes, exercise tools and meetings have made it the leading weight control company in the world.

Weight Watchers' Points System: How Does It Work?

Weight Watchers is the first company to introduce a weight loss program that goes beyond dieting and calorie counting: it assigns points to food items and dishes that will help you control your calories and keep track of what you eat on a daily basis.

Upon becoming a member of Weight Watchers, a person will be assigned a daily point allowance based on personal figures such as age, height and weight. Once the daily point allocation has been computed, he/she must eat meals during this day that will not exceed his/her allowed points. By doing so, the individual is able to lose weight and enjoy good food at the same time.

The former PointsPlus system assigned points for food based on broad categories such as protein, fat, carbohydrates and calories. But with the new SmartPoints system, specific components are used to have a more realistic measure of the food item in terms of its nutritive effect on weight loss.

Features of New SmartPoints System

The new SmartPoints program uses four major nutrients when computing for the points of a specific food or meal, namely:

- Calories;
- Sugar;
- Saturated Fat; and
- Protein

The science behind this new system is simple: if you eat more protein, the lesser SmartPoints you consume and the faster you are able to lose weight. On the other hand, if you choose to eat sweets or unhealthy fats which have higher SmartPoints values, you will quickly deplete your daily point allocation. Moreover, you may find yourself craving for more food and eating more than you should. This is the reason why foods that have higher SmartPoints values tend to slow down the weight loss process.

In conclusion, the goal of the new SmartPoints system is to provide you with the right tools and know-how to choose nutritious dishes that are lower in points. These foods consist of healthier ingredients such as fruits, vegetables, lean protein, low-fat dairy and other organic items.   Eating low SmartPoints foods daily while engaging in exercise and social activities helps create a healthy weight loss regimen and a better quality of life.

The following chapter will show you how to compute food points in the new SmartPoints program.

Chapter 2 Knowing Your Weight Watcher Figures

"If you're going to lose weight, you have to do it by changing your way of thinking about food. It cannot be the highlight of your life."

Jean Nidetch
Businesswoman and Founder, Weight Watchers

The new SmartPoints system is a more credible way of assigning points to everyday meals. It takes into consideration vital nutrients, namely protein, sugar, saturated fat and calories, which are all key players in the weight loss process. Luckily, a lot of cookbooks and recipe websites contain nutritional information that will enable us to compute the SmartPoints value of your chosen dish.

Knowing Your Daily SmartPoints Allowance

The first step towards reaching your fitness goals with the SmartPoints system is to determine your Weight Watchers daily point allowance. Upon signing up with the program, the company provides you with your daily point allocation based on the following categories:

- Gender;
- Age;
- Height;
- Weight; and
- Daily Activity Level

If you are a non-member of Weight Watchers but want to know your daily SmartPoints allowance, there is an online Weight Watchers calculator on the website www.calculator.net that will help you determine your number.

Computing a Meal's SmartPoints

Once you know your daily point allowance, you may now start computing for SmartPoints. Weight Watchers provides a variety of online tools to help their members determine the food points of their favorite meals. Moreover, a Weight Watchers SmartPoints Calculator can be purchased from both the organization and Amazon.com to help you keep track of your daily points balance.

However, if you are not a member of Weight Watchers but still want to try out the

SmartPoints program for yourself, you can still calculate the points of a specific recipe using the following formula:

$$\frac{\text{Calories} + (\text{Sugar X 4}) + (\text{Saturated Fat X 9}) - (3.2 \text{ x Protein})}{33}$$

As shown in the formula, points are added for the components that cause weight gain while points are subtracted for protein, a nutrient that promotes metabolism, fat loss and muscle formation. You can also try visiting the website www.calculatorcat.com for an online version of the SmartPoints calculator.

Life-Changing Benefits of Low SmartPoints Meals

Over the years, several studies done by the British Medical Journal, American Journal of Medicine and American Dietetic Association have proven how the Weight Watchers method of calculating food points have resulted in more weight loss success stories than other diet programs.

Here are the major benefits of eating low SmartPoints meals in terms of weight management and improving one's quality of life:

- Foods that are low in SmartPoints contain fewer calories, carbs and sugar, thus weight loss is consequently achieved;

- The SmartPoints system is healthier and more sustainable as it discourages crash dieting or skipping meals;

- High protein and vitamin content of low SmartPoints foods lead to prolonged feelings of fullness, thus preventing unnecessary cravings or binge eating that are huge factors in weight gain;

- As you become used to calculating points, an increased appreciation for nutritional values and natural flavors is developed within you; and

- A lot of cookbooks and recipe sites include nutritional information as well as SmartPoints values for each dish, thus making healthy meal preparation more convenient.

Now that you have determined your Weight Watcher daily points allocation number, it is now time to start enjoying food and losing weight at the same time. Luckily for you, this book contains 50 SmartPoints dinner recipes that are low on points but high on flavors and healthier nutrients. These mouth-watering recipes will not only satisfy your taste buds but will likewise help you reach your fitness goals.

Chapter 3 Salad Recipes

Spicy Kale Salad with Lemon Vinaigrette

Ingredients:

- 8 cups kale leaves

- 3 tablespoons olive oil

- 3 tablespoons lemon juice

- 2 teaspoons chili powder

- 1 teaspoon sea salt

- 1 teaspoon garlic powder

Directions:

1. Whisk olive oil and lemon juice in a large bowl until smooth. Season the vinaigrette with chili powder, garlic powder and salt.

2. Add in the kale leaves and toss them together. Place the salad in the fridge and chill for 1 hour. Serve cold.

3. This recipe makes 5 servings.

Nutrition: 130 calories; 0g sugar; 1g saturated fat; 6g protein; 19g carbohydrates; 4g fiber

Smart Points: 4

Old-Fashioned Greek Salad

Ingredients:

- 5 cups romaine lettuce

- 1 red onion, peeled and thinly-sliced

- 2 cups cherry tomatoes, halved

- 2 cups diced cucumbers

- 2 cups pitted olives, halved

- 1 teaspoon chopped fresh basil

- ¾ cup feta cheese, crumbled

- 1 cup balsamic salad dressing

Directions:

1. Place romaine lettuce, onions, tomatoes, cucumbers and olives in a salad bowl then toss. Set aside.

2. Whisk together basil and salad dressing. Pour the salad dressing into the vegetables then toss until the greens are well-coated. Chill the salad in the fridge for 30 minutes.

3. After 30 minutes, take out the salad from the fridge. Sprinkle the feta

cheese on top of it then serve immediately.

4. This recipe makes 4 servings.

Nutrition: 194 calories; 11g sugar; 4g saturated fat; 9g protein; 17g carbohydrates; 4g fiber

Smart Points: 7

Spicy Corn and Black Bean Salad

Ingredients:

- ½ red bell pepper, deseeded and sliced thinly

- ½ cup canned corn kernels, drained

- ½ cup cherry tomato halves

- ½ cup canned black beans, drained

- 4 tablespoons chopped cilantro

- 2 teaspoons olive oil

- 3 teaspoons lemon juice

- ½ teaspoon chili powder

- Pinch of sea salt and black pepper

Directions:

1. Place the bell pepper, corn, tomatoes, black beans and cilantro in a bowl then toss. Set aside.

2. In a separate bowl, whisk together olive oil, lemon juice, chili powder, salt and black pepper. Pour the dressing on top of the salad then toss them together. Transfer the salad to

individual dinner plates and serve immediately.

3. This recipe makes 2 servings.

Nutrition: 137 calories; 5g sugar; 1g saturated fat; 6g protein; 24g carbohydrates; 7g fiber

Smart Points: 4

Tuna, Apple and Cranberry Salad

Ingredients:

- 300 grams canned tuna in water, drained

- 6 tablespoons dried cranberries

- 1 cup diced apples

- 1 ½ cups chopped lettuce

- ½ cup chopped celery

- 2 tablespoons lemon juice

- 1 tablespoon dill

- 6 tablespoons light mayonnaise

- Pinch of salt and black pepper

Directions:

1. Whisk together mayonnaise, dill, lemon juice, salt and pepper in a large bowl. Add in tuna, cranberries, apples and celery then toss.

2. Place the chopped lettuce on smaller plates then spoon the salad on top of it. Serve immediately.

3. This recipe makes 4 servings.

Nutrition: 205 calories; 11g sugar; 1g saturated fat; 17g protein; 18g carbohydrates; 2g fiber

Smart Points: 6

Mediterranean Vegetable Salad with Lime Dressing

Ingredients:

- 1 summer squash, peeled and julienned
- 1 medium cucumber, peeled and julienned
- ½ green bell pepper, deseeded and sliced thinly
- ½ cup pitted black olives, halved
- 1 carrot, peeled and julienned
- ½ red onion, peeled and chopped
- 1 tablespoon chopped cilantro
- 2 tablespoons lime juice
- 1 tablespoon olive oil
- Pinch of salt and black pepper

Directions:

1. Pour the lime juice and olive oil in a salad bowl then whisk. Season it with salt and pepper while whisking the dressing.

2. Mix in the summer squash, cucumber, bell pepper, carrot, cilantro and red onion with the dressing. Gently toss the ingredients together then let it chill in the fridge for 1 hour. Serve cold.

3. This recipe makes 4 servings.

Nutrition: 72 calories; 6g sugar; 0g saturated fat; 2g protein; 10g carbohydrates; 3g fiber

Smart Points: 2

Peach Arugula Salad with Balsamic Dressing

Ingredients:

- 3 peaches, peeled, pitted and sliced

- 120 grams arugula leaves

- 1 small red onion, peeled and chopped

- 1 medium tomato, chopped

- 100 grams goat cheese

- 1 tablespoon balsamic vinegar

- 3 tablespoons olive oil

- 1 teaspoon mustard

- ½ tablespoon honey

- ½ teaspoon sea salt

- ½ teaspoon white pepper

Directions:

1. Whisk together balsamic vinegar, olive oil, mustard, honey, sea salt and white pepper until the dressing

is smooth. Chill it in the fridge for 30 minutes.

2. Place the arugula, peaches, onion, tomato and goat cheese in a salad bowl. Pour the balsamic dressing on the vegetables then toss them together. Serve the salad in smaller dinner plates.

3. This recipe makes 5 servings.

Nutrition: 180 calories; 9g sugar; 5g saturated fat; 6g protein; 11g carbohydrates; 2g fiber

Smart Points: 7

Zesty Potato and Cucumber Salad with Dijon Mayo

Ingredients:

- 5 medium white potatoes, peeled and cubed

- 1 medium cucumber, peeled and thinly-sliced

- 1 tablespoon grated carrots

- ½ sweet onion, minced

- ½ cup organic mayonnaise

- 1 teaspoon sea salt

- 1 ½ teaspoons Dijon mustard

- ½ teaspoon ground black pepper

Directions:

1. Place the potatoes in a pot filled with water then place it over high flame. Cover the pot then wait for the water to boil. Once the water is boiling, lower the flame to medium-high then cook the potatoes for 15 minutes or until they are tender. Drain the

potatoes then place them in a bowl to cool. Set aside.

2. While the potatoes are cooling, make the salad dressing by whisking together the mayonnaise, sea salt, mustard and black pepper.

3. Add the cucumbers, carrots and sweet onions into the bowl of potatoes and mix. Pour in the dressing then toss gently. Refrigerate the salad for 2-3 hours. Serve cold.

4. This recipe makes 4 servings.

Nutrition: 185 calories; 3g sugar; 2g saturated fat; 2g protein; 21g carbohydrates; 2g fiber

Smart Points: 6

Spinach, Arugula and Chicken Salad

Ingredients:

- 3 cups spinach leaves

- 2 cups arugula leaves

- 2 small boneless and skinless chicken breast halves

- 1 ¼ cups frozen blueberries, drained and roughly chopped

- ¼ cup chopped toasted almonds

- ¼ cup apple cider vinegar

- 2 tablespoons honey

- ¼ cup olive oil

- Pinch of salt and black pepper

Directions:

1. Brown the chicken breasts on a grill pan for 6-8 minutes per side. Once the chicken is cooked, place it on a chopping board then dice it. Place the diced meat in a salad bowl and set aside.

2. In a separate bowl, whisk together honey, apple cider vinegar, olive oil, chopped almonds, salt, pepper and ¼ cup of the blueberries. Pour the dressing on top of the diced chicken.

3. Add the spinach, arugula and remaining blueberries into the salad bowl then toss gently until the greens and chicken are evenly-coated. Serve the salad on individual dinner plates.

4. This recipe makes 4 servings.

Nutrition: 266 calories; 14g sugar; 3g saturated fat; 11g protein; 18g carbohydrates; 3g fiber

Smart Points: 9

Curried Cauliflower and Quinoa Salad

Ingredients:

- 2 cups cauliflower florets

- 2 cups pre-cooked quinoa

- 1 ½ teaspoon curry powder

- ½ teaspoon minced ginger

- 2 tablespoons olive oil

- 1 tablespoon lemon juice

- ½ cup pomegranate seeds

- 1 teaspoon minced garlic

- Pinch of salt and black pepper

Directions:

1. Place the cauliflower florets in a bowl then add in 1 tablespoon of olive oil, curry powder, ginger and garlic. Toss the florets until well-coated. Place the vegetables on a parchment-lined baking sheet then roast it in a 400°F oven for 15-20 minutes.

2. Take the roasted vegetables from the oven then transfer it to a salad bowl. Let it cool for 10 minutes.

3. In a separate bowl, whisk together the lemon juice, pomegranate seeds, salt, pepper and remaining olive oil. Pour the dressing on top of the roasted cauliflower then mix in the quinoa. Gently toss the salad then serve immediately.

Nutrition: 177 calories; 5g sugar; 1g saturated fat; 6g protein; 26g carbohydrates; 4g fiber

Smart Points: 4

Scrumptious Taco Salad with Sour Cream

Ingredients:

- 1 cup lean ground turkey

- 8 cups shredded iceberg lettuce

- ½ cup thinly-sliced red onion

- 1 red bell pepper, deseeded and chopped

- 4 tablespoons canned corn kernels

- ½ cup canned black beans, drained

- 6 tortilla chips, crushed

- 2 teaspoons taco seasoning

- 4 tablespoons salsa

- 3 tablespoons sour cream

- 1 teaspoon olive oil

Directions:

1. Heat the olive oil in a pan over medium-high flame. Add the onion and bell pepper to the hot oil and cook for 4 minutes.

2. Add the turkey and taco seasoning into the pan and continue cooking the taco mixture for 6-8 minutes. Once the turkey is cooked, pour in the corn and black beans and stir. Let the mixture cook for another 4 minutes then turn off the flame.

3. Place the shredded lettuce on a serving platter then top it with the crushed tortilla chips. Pour the cooked taco mixture on top of the chips, followed by the salsa then finally, the sour cream. Serve immediately.

4. This recipe makes 3 servings.

Nutrition: 354 calories; 11g sugar; 4g saturated fat; 31g protein; 37g carbohydrates; 9g fiber

Smart Points: 7

Chapter 4 Soup and Chowder Recipes

Chunky Vegetable and Chicken Soup

Ingredients:

- 1 large boneless and skinless chicken breast, boiled

- 3 cups chicken stock

- 1 small red onion, chopped

- 1 ¾ cup canned cannellini beans, drained

- 2 cups shredded cabbage

- 1 ½ cups stewed tomatoes

- 1 large carrot, peeled and diced

- 1 cup frozen green peas, thawed

- ½ teaspoon salt

- Pinch of black pepper

- 1 teaspoon olive oil

Directions:

1. Using two forks, shred the boiled chicken breast into flakes and set aside.

2. Heat the olive oil in a large pot over medium-high flame. Add the onions to the pot and cook until translucent. Next, add in carrots and cannellini beans then stir while cooking for 5 minutes.

3. Add in the green peas, stewed tomatoes and shredded chicken to the pot and let it cook for 5 minutes. Pour in the chicken stock then season the soup with salt and pepper. Cover the pot and lower the flame to medium. Simmer the soup for 10 minutes.

4. After 10 minutes, add the cabbage into the soup then stir. Cook the soup for another 10 minutes with constant stirring.

5. Pour the soup into smaller bowls and serve immediately.

6. This recipe makes 8-10 servings.

Nutrition: 150 calories; 5g sugar; 0.5g saturated fat; 21g protein; 15g carbohydrates; 4g fiber

Smart Points: 2

Low-Calorie Butternut Soup

Ingredients:

- 4 cups diced fresh butternut squash

- 4 cups chicken stock

- 1 celery stalk, chopped

- 1 yellow onion, minced

- 1 cup diced carrots

- ½ teaspoon chopped thyme

- 2 tablespoons olive oil

- Pinch of salt and black pepper

Directions:

1. Heat the oil in a pot over medium-high flame. Add the onion, carrots, celery to the hot oil and cook them for 4 minutes. Add the butternut squash cubes, salt, pepper, thyme and chicken stock. Stir while cooking for 5 minutes.

2. Cover the pot and bring the soup to a boil. Lower the flame to medium then let the soup simmer for 30

minutes. Poke the squash with a fork: once it is soft and tender, turn off the heat.

3. Pour the soup into a blender then puree it. Serve it while hot.

4. This recipe makes 4 servings.

Nutrition: 140 calories; 4g sugar; 1g saturated fat; 6g protein; 20g carbohydrates; 5g fiber

Smart Points: 4

Buttery Cream of Corn Soup

Ingredients:

- 4 ears fresh corn, kernels sliced off from corn cobs

- 1 cup skim milk

- 1½ teaspoons butter

- 2 garlic cloves, minced

- ½ sweet onion, minced

- 2 cups chicken broth

- ½ cup heavy cream

- ¾ cup canned evaporated milk

- 1 ½ teaspoons olive oil

- ½ teaspoon salt

Directions:

1. Place the butter, olive oil, garlic and onions in a pot over medium-high flame and sauté the spices for 5 minutes. Lower the flame to medium then add in the corn kernels. Continue sautéing the ingredients for

4 minutes while seasoning them with salt.

2. Add in the skim milk, evaporated milk and empty corn cobs. Pour in the broth then cover the pot. Let the chowder simmer for 1 hour.

3. After 1 hour, remove the cobs from the chowder then mix in the heavy cream. Turn off the heat then pour the soup into individual bowls. Serve immediately.

4. This recipe makes 4 servings.

Nutrition: 237 calories; 20g sugar; 2g saturated fat; 11g protein; 41g carbohydrates; 3g fiber

Smart Points: 9

Quick and Easy Tomato and Zucchini Soup

Ingredients:

- 1 ¾ cups chopped tomatoes

- 220 grams sliced zucchini

- ½ green bell pepper, deseeded and chopped

- ½ cup chopped celery

- ¼ cup minced onion

- 2 garlic cloves, minced

- 100 grams Italian sausage

- 1 ½ cups chicken stock

- ½ teaspoon chili powder

- Pinch of salt and black pepper

Directions:

1. Cook the sausage in a saucepan over medium-high flame for 5 minutes. Add in the garlic, onion, celery and bell pepper. Continue cooking for 3-4 minutes or until the sausage has browned.

2. Add in the zucchini, tomatoes and broth then stir. Season the soup with salt and pepper. Cover the pot and let the soup simmer for 10 minutes.

3. Stir the soup then pour it into individual bowls. Serve immediately.

4. This recipe makes 3 servings.

Nutrition: 133 calories; 6g sugar; 1g saturated fat; 11g protein; 12g carbohydrates; 2g fiber

Smart Points: 3

Cheesy Broccoli Chowder

Ingredients:

- 2 cups broccoli florets, roughly chopped
- 1 small carrot, peeled and chopped
- ½ cup chopped celery
- 1 small onion, minced
- 3 garlic cloves, minced
- 1 cup grated Parmesan cheese
- ½ cup canned evaporated milk
- 2 teaspoons olive oil
- 4 cups chicken stock
- Pinch of salt and black pepper

Directions:

1. Heat the olive oil in a saucepan over medium-high flame. Add the garlic, onion, carrots and celery to the hot oil and cook for 5 minutes. Once the vegetables are tender, add in the broccoli then stir.

2. Pour the chicken stock into the saucepan then stir. Lower the flame to medium then cover the pot. Allow the soup to simmer for 10 minutes.

3. After 10 minutes, turn off the flame then mix in the cheese and milk. Stir continuously until the cheese melts. Pour the soup mixture into a blender and process until the desired consistency is met.

4. Transfer the soup to individual bowls and serve while hot.

5. This recipe makes 4 servings.

Nutrition: 238 calories; 8g sugar; 7g saturated fat; 14g protein; 13g carbohydrates; 4g fiber

Smart Points: 6

Oven-Roasted Pepper and Tomato Soup

Ingredients:

- 2 medium tomatoes

- 2 Serrano peppers

- 2 cups canned corn kernels

- 1 teaspoon minced garlic

- ½ tablespoon minced onions

- 2 cups vegetable stock

- ¼ teaspoon cumin

- ½ teaspoon paprika

- 1 teaspoon olive oil

- Pinch of salt and black pepper

Directions:

1. Place the tomatoes and peppers on a parchment-lined baking sheet. Drizzle the vegetables with ½ teaspoon of olive oil then season it with pepper and salt. Roast it in a 400°F oven for 15 minutes.

2. After 15 minutes, remove the veggies from the oven then remove their stems and outer skin. Set aside.

3. Heat the remaining olive oil in a saucepan over medium-high flame. Add the garlic and onions to the pot and sauté for 3 minutes. Gradually add in the paprika and cumin then cook for a few more seconds.

4. Once the spices are fragrant, add the tomatoes, peppers and corn into the saucepan and stir for 5 minutes. Pour in the stock then cover the pot. Let the soup simmer for 15 minutes then turn off the flame.

5. Using an immersion blender, process the soup until it becomes creamy. Pour it into smaller bowls and serve immediately.

6. This recipe makes 3 servings.

Nutrition: 100 calories; 10g sugar; 0g saturated fat; 3g protein; 19g carbohydrates; 4g fiber

Smart Points: 4

Creamy Asparagus Chowder

Ingredients:

- 450 grams asparagus, trimmed and chopped into 1-inch pieces

- 1 white potato, peeled and diced

- 1 leek, chopped into 1-inch pieces

- 1 tablespoon chopped chives

- 4 cups chicken broth

- 1 tablespoon butter

- ½ cup sour cream

- Pinch of salt and black pepper

Directions:

1. Melt the butter in a saucepan over medium-high flame. Add the leeks to the pot and cook for 8 minutes. Mix in the potatoes and let it cook for 5 minutes. Pour the broth into the saucepan and cover it. Let the soup come to a boil.

2. Once the soup is boiling, lower the flame to medium then add in the

asparagus. Stir the soup then allow it to simmer for 10 minutes or until the potatoes are tender.

3. Pour the soup into a blender then process it until a smooth and creamy texture is reached. Place the soup back into the saucepan then mix in sour cream and chives. Serve the soup in smaller bowls while hot.

4. This recipe makes 4 servings.

Nutrition: 140 calories; 6g sugar; 3g saturated fat; 5g protein; 19g carbohydrates; 3g fiber

Smart Points: 5

Rosemary Cauliflower Soup

Ingredients:

- 400 grams cauliflower florets

- ½ teaspoon dried rosemary

- ½ cup chopped celery

- 1 sweet onion, minced

- 4 cups vegetable stock

- 1 ½ tablespoons olive oil

- Pinch of salt and black pepper

Directions:

1. Lay the cauliflower florets in a baking sheet lined with tin foil. Pour a tablespoon of olive oil all over the veggies then season it with salt and pepper. Roast the florets in a 400°F oven for 25 minutes. Once the florets are tender, turn off the oven and let them cool at room temperature.

2. Heat the remaining olive oil in a saucepan over medium-high flame then sauté both the onions and celery for 4 minutes. Add in the roasted

cauliflower and continue cooking the veggies for 5 minutes.

3. Slowly pour in the stock then sprinkle the rosemary into the soup. Lower the flame to medium and let the soup simmer for 15 minutes. After 15 minutes, remove the saucepan from the flame then puree the soup with an immersion blender.

4. Place the saucepan back onto the stovetop and let the soup simmer for an extra 5 minutes. Stir constantly. Pour the soup into individual bowls and serve immediately.

5. This recipe makes 4 servings.

Nutrition: 231 calories; 7g sugar; 1g saturated fat; 8g protein; 35g carbohydrates; 7g fiber

Smart Points: 7

Vegetarian Minestrone

Ingredients:

- 4 cups low-sodium vegetable stock
- 2 cups cooked elbow macaroni
- 1 ¾ cups canned navy beans, pureed
- 1 cup diced carrots
- 3 cups chopped tomatoes
- 1 sweet onion, minced
- 1 teaspoon minced garlic
- ½ cup chopped celery
- 1 medium zucchini, diced
- 2 tablespoons chopped basil
- 1 teaspoon chopped fresh rosemary
- 2 cups spinach leaves, chopped
- 2 teaspoons olive oil
- ½ cup grated Parmesan cheese
- Pinch of salt and black pepper

Directions:

1. Heat the oil in a pan over medium-high flame. Add in the garlic, onions, carrots and celery. Let the veggies cook for 10 minutes then transfer these to a slow cooker.

2. Add the pureed beans, tomatoes, basil and vegetable stock into the slow cooker. Season the soup with salt, rosemary and pepper. Cover the pot and let it cook on low for 6 hours.

3. After 6 hours, add the zucchini and spinach into the minestrone and stir. Cover and continue cooking it for 30 minutes. After 30 minutes, transfer the minestrone to a serving bowl then mix in the cooked macaroni. Sprinkle parmesan cheese on top then serve immediately.

4. This recipe makes 8 servings.

Nutrition: 190 calories; 4g sugar; 2g saturated fat; 9g protein; 32g carbohydrates; 8g fiber

Smart Points: 4

Freezer-Friendly Mushroom Soup

Ingredients:

- 2 cups chopped white mushrooms
- 1 cup vegetable broth
- 2 garlic cloves, minced
- 1 tablespoon fresh thyme
- ½ cup skim milk
- ½ cup canned evaporated milk
- 1½ teaspoons butter
- ¾ teaspoon Worcestershire sauce
- ½ cup skim milk
- Pinch of nutmeg
- Pinch of salt and black pepper

Directions:

1. Heat the olive oil and butter in a saucepan over medium-high flame. Add the garlic and sauté until golden brown. Mix in the mushrooms, Worcestershire sauce and thyme then cook for 15 minutes.

2. Once the mushrooms have dried up, pour the vegetable broth into the saucepan and stir. Bring to a boil then lower the flame. Season the soup with salt, pepper and nutmeg then let it simmer for 10 minutes.

3. After 10 minutes, mix in the skim milk and evaporated milk then simmer it for 2 minutes. Turn off the flame then let it cool for 10 minutes. Pour the soup into individual bowls and serve warm.

4. If you want to store extra batches, let the soup cool completely then place it in an airtight container. Place it in the freezer for future use.

Nutrition: 137 calories; 13g sugar; 2g saturated fat; 9g protein; 16g carbohydrates; 1g fiber

Smart Points: 6

Chapter 5 Chicken & Turkey Recipes

Crispy Baked Chicken Nuggets

Ingredients:

- 2 medium boneless and skinless chicken cutlets, diced into 10 cubes

- ¼ cup panko breadcrumbs

- ½ cup all-purpose flour

- 1 large egg, whisked

- ½ teaspoon garlic powder

- ¼ teaspoon onion powder

- ½ teaspoon salt

- Pinch of white pepper

Directions:

1. Preheat the oven to 375°F and line a baking sheet with parchment paper.

2. Combine breadcrumbs, salt, pepper, onion powder and garlic powder. Set aside.

3. Dredge the chicken pieces into the flour. Next, dip each piece into the whisked egg then roll it on the breadcrumb mixture until the sides are evenly-coated. Place the nuggets on the lined baking sheet.

4. Bake the chicken nuggets for 8 minutes. After 8 minutes, flip them over then finish baking them for 6-7 minutes. Place the nuggets on a wire rack to cool. Serve warm.

5. This recipe makes 2 servings (5 nuggets per serving).

Nutrition: 180 calories; 1g sugar; 0.5g saturated fat; 28g protein; 8g carbohydrates; 1g fiber

Smart Points: 3

Juicy Turkey Burgers with Zucchini Salsa

Ingredients:

- 450 grams lean ground turkey

- ½ cup breadcrumbs

- 1 egg, whisked

- 2 garlic cloves, minced

- ½ red onion, minced

- 2 tablespoons chopped parsley

- ½ teaspoon black pepper

- ½ teaspoon sea salt

- 1 tablespoon olive oil

- 1 medium zucchini, peeled and diced

- 2 tablespoons lime juice

- ½ cup chopped green onions

- ¼ teaspoon salt

- 1 medium tomato, diced

Directions:

1. To make the burger, mix together the turkey meat, egg, breadcrumbs, garlic and onions. Season the patty mixture with salt and pepper. Form this into 4 burgers and set aside.

2. Heat the olive oil in a pan over medium-high flame. Once the oil is hot, place the burgers on the pan and cook each side for 5-7 minutes.

3. While the burgers are cooking, mix together the zucchini, tomatoes, lime juice, salt and green onions.

4. Once the burgers are cooked, transfer them to individual dinner plates. Serve each burger patty with a side of the zucchini salsa.

5. This recipe makes 4 servings.

Nutrition: 314 calories; 3g sugar; 4g saturated fat; 26g protein; 15g carbohydrates; 2g fiber

Smart Points: 8

Grilled Chicken in Red Wine Sauce

Ingredients:

- 2 boneless and skinless chicken breast cutlets

- 2 tablespoons red wine

- 1 cup button mushrooms, sliced

- 2 tablespoons chicken broth

- 1 teaspoon all-purpose flour

- 1 teaspoon olive oil

- Pinch of salt and black pepper

Directions:

1. Moisten a grill pan with some cooking spray then place it on the stove over medium-high flame. Lay the chicken cutlets on the grill and brown each side for 8 minutes. Place the cutlets on a plate and set aside.

2. Heat the oil in a skillet over medium flame. Add the mushrooms into the hot oil and sauté for 2-3 minutes. Mix in the salt, pepper and flour then stir constantly. Finally, pour in the

broth and red wine. Cover the skillet and let the mixture simmer and thicken.

3. Once the sauce has thickened, turn off the flame and stir it for a few seconds. Pour the mushrooms and sauce over the chicken and serve immediately.

4. This recipe makes 2 servings.

Nutrition: 231 calories; 1g sugar; 1g saturated fat; 27g protein; 5g carbohydrates; 1g fiber

Smart Points: 4

Sweet and Spicy Turkey Cutlets

Ingredients:

- 4 medium-sized turkey breast cutlets
- 2 tablespoons maple syrup
- 3 teaspoons hot sauce
- 2 tablespoons lime juice
- 2 garlic cloves, minced
- 2 tablespoons low-sodium soy sauce
- 2 teaspoons apple cider vinegar
- 1 tablespoon olive oil

Directions:

1. Combine the maple syrup, hot sauce, lime juice, garlic, soy sauce and vinegar in a mixing bowl. Place the turkey breasts inside the bowl and let it marinade overnight.

2. Heat the oil in a grill pan over medium high flame. Place the marinated turkey breasts onto the pan then cook each side for 3 minutes or until grill marks appear.

Place the turkey cutlets on a large plate and serve immediately.

3. This recipe makes 4 servings.

Nutrition: 210 calories; 10g sugar; 0g saturated fat; 33g protein; 11g carbohydrates; 0g fiber

Smart Points: 5

Sesame-Crusted Chicken Fingers

Ingredients:

- 450 grams boneless and skinless chicken strips
- 2 tablespoons all-purpose flour
- 2 tablespoons toasted sesame seeds
- 1 tablespoon soy sauce
- 1 tablespoon water
- 1 tablespoon dry sherry
- 1 teaspoon minced ginger
- 1 tablespoon honey
- 2 teaspoons olive oil
- ½ teaspoon five-spice powder
- Pinch of salt and black pepper

Directions:

1. In a small bowl, whisk together soy sauce, water, sherry, ginger, honey, and five-spice powder. Set aside.

2. Place the chicken strips in a bowl then add in flour, salt and pepper.

Toss until the chicken pieces are evenly-coated.

3. Heat the oil in a pan over medium-high flame. Once the oil is hot, add the chicken strips and cook for 5 minutes or until the sides have turned light brown. Lower the flame to medium, pour in the soy mixture and stir. Let the chicken and sauce cook together for 3 minutes or until the sauce has reduced.

4. Turn off the flame then roll the chicken strips one-by-one on the toasted sesame seeds. Place them on a serving plate.

5. This recipe makes 4 servings.

Nutrition: 216 calories; 3g sugar; 1g saturated fat; 28g protein; 8g carbohydrates; 1g fiber

Smart Points: 4

Shredded Turkey with BBQ Applesauce

Ingredients:

- 450 grams boneless and skinless turkey cutlets

- ½ sweet onion, minced

- ¼ cup unsweetened applesauce

- 1 apple, peeled, cored and sliced

- ¼ cup chicken stock

- ½ cup barbecue sauce

- 1 garlic clove, minced

- ½ teaspoon cumin

- ¼ teaspoon black pepper

- ½ teaspoon chili powder

- ½ teaspoon salt

Directions:

1. Whisk together the applesauce, chicken stock, barbecue sauce, garlic, black pepper, chili powder, cumin and salt in a bowl. Set aside.

2. Lay the turkey cutlets, onions and apple slices inside a crock pot. Pour the applesauce mixture into the pot then cover it. Cook the dish on low heat for 3-4 hours or until tender.

3. Shred the turkey into long strands by using a pair of forks. Transfer the shredded meat on a serving platter then pour the remaining juices on top of it. Serve immediately.

4. This recipe makes 4 servings.

Nutrition: 215 calories; 15g sugar; 1g saturated fat; 25g protein; 22g carbohydrates; 2g fiber

Smart Points: 4

Soft Chicken Tacos with Cheese Sauce

Ingredients:

- 450 grams boneless and skinless chicken breasts

- 3 pieces jalapeno peppers, chopped

- 1 teaspoon olive oil

- ½ teaspoon oregano

- 1 teaspoon taco seasoning

- ½ teaspoon garlic powder

- Pinch of salt and black pepper

- ¼ cup plain yoghurt

- ¼ cup cream cheese

- 2 tablespoons chopped cilantro

- 1 tablespoon cayenne pepper

- 6 corn tortillas

Directions:

1. Boil the chicken in salted water until fully-cooked. Drain the water from the meat then place the chicken on a

plate. Shred the chicken meat then set aside.

2. Heat the oil in a pan over medium-high flame. Add the shredded chicken into the pan then season it with salt, pepper, garlic powder, oregano and taco seasoning. Gradually mix in the jalapenos and stir while cooking for 5 minutes. Turn off the flame and set aside.

3. In a separate bowl, whisk together the yoghurt, cream cheese, cilantro and cayenne pepper. This will serve as the sauce inside the taco.

4. Warm the tortillas on the stove. Place a tortilla on a plate then spoon a generous amount of chicken and cheese sauce on top of it. Fold the tortilla in half then serve immediately.

5. This recipe makes 3 servings.

Nutrition:

Smart Points: 7

Easy Chicken and Broccoli Stir-Fry

Ingredients:

- 3 large boneless and skinless chicken breasts, diced

- 2 cups broccoli florets

- 2 garlic cloves, minced

- 1 sweet onion, minced

- 1 tablespoon chopped fresh basil

- 1 teaspoon oregano

- ½ cup chicken stock

- Pinch of salt and black pepper

- 1 tablespoon olive oil

Directions:

1. Heat the olive oil in a pan over medium flame. Add the garlic and onions to the hot oil and sauté until the onions are translucent. Mix in the broccoli and chicken pieces and stir-fry for 5 minutes.

2. Pour the chicken stock into the pan then season the dish with salt, pepper, basil and oregano. Cover the pan and let it simmer for 4 minutes or until the liquid has evaporated. Serve immediately.

3. This recipe makes 4 servings.

Nutrition: 388 calories; 4g sugar; 2g saturated fat; 59g protein; 14g carbohydrates; 5g fiber

Smart Points: 7

Hot and Spicy Turkey and Lentil Chili

Ingredients:

- 220 grams lean ground turkey
- 1 red bell pepper, deseeded and diced
- 200 grams dry lentils
- ¾ cup tomato sauce
- 1 small red onion, minced
- 3 ¼ cup chicken stock
- 2 tablespoons minced garlic
- ¾ teaspoon paprika
- ¾ teaspoon chili seasoning
- 1 teaspoon onion powder
- Pinch of salt and black pepper
- 1 teaspoon olive oil

Directions:

1. Heat the olive oil in a pan over high flame. Brown the ground turkey in the hot oil then turn off the flame.

Transfer the ground meat into the slow cooker.

2. Add the lentils, bell peppers, onion, garlic, and tomato sauce into the slow cooker then stir. Season the ingredients with paprika, onion powder, salt, pepper and chili seasoning.

3. Cover the pot then cook the chili on low for 7 hours. Stir every hour so the meat is evenly-cooked. Serve hot.

4. This recipe makes 5 servings.

Nutrition: 318 calories; 5g sugar; 1g saturated fat; 32g protein; 42g carbohydrates; 19g fiber

Smart Points: 6

Spicy Turkey and Cashew Dinner

Ingredients:

- 580 grams boneless and skinless turkey breast, sliced into strips

- ¼ cup toasted cashews, chopped

- 4 garlic cloves, minced

- 1 onion, peeled and chopped

- 1 red bell pepper, deseeded and julienned

- 2 tablespoons chopped green onions

- 1 tablespoon minced ginger

- 3 tablespoons oyster sauce

- ½ cup chicken stock

- 1 tablespoon honey

- 2 tablespoons soy sauce

- 1 tablespoon olive oil

Directions:

1. Heat the oil in a skillet over medium-high flame. Sauté the garlic, ginger and onions until the onions become

translucent. Add in the turkey strips and cook for 3 minutes.

2. Pour the stock over the chicken and let it simmer for 5 minutes. Once most of the stock has evaporated, add in the bell pepper and continue cooking for 2 minutes.

3. After 2 minutes, add in the oyster sauce, honey and soy sauce. Stir-fry the dish for a few more minutes then turn off the flame. Transfer the dish to a serving plate then sprinkle the cashew and green onions on top. Serve immediately.

4. This recipe makes 4 servings.

Nutrition: 314 calories; 7g sugar; 1g saturated fat; 36g protein; 18g carbohydrates; 2g fiber

Smart Points: 6

Chapter 6 Beef & Pork Recipes

Sweet Balsamic Pork Medallions

Ingredients:

- 450 grams pork tenderloin

- 1 tablespoon soy sauce

- 2 tablespoons balsamic vinegar

- 1 ½ tablespoons brown sugar

- ¼ cup vegetable stock

- ¼ teaspoon garlic powder

- ½ teaspoon chili powder

- ¼ teaspoon cumin

- Pinch of salt and black pepper

Directions:

1. In a medium bowl, mix together brown sugar, garlic powder, chili powder, cumin, salt and pepper. Place the tenderloin into the spice bowl and rub the spices all over the

meat. Arrange the spiced pork inside your slow cooker.

2. Pour the vinegar, soy sauce and vegetable stock into the pot. Cover it then set the temperature to low. Cook the tenderloin for 6 hours.

3. After 6 hours, transfer the tenderloin on a chopping board and slice it into half-inch thick medallions. Arrange the pork slices on a serving plate then drizzle the juices from the pot on top of it. Serve immediately.

4. This recipe makes 3 servings.

Nutrition: 208 calories, 9g sugar; 1g saturated fat; 32g protein; 9g carbohydrates; 0g fiber

Smart Points: 4

Shredded Beef Stew

Ingredients:

- 700 grams beef top round, fat trimmed off

- 2 ½ teaspoons Worcestershire sauce

- 3 cups chicken stock

- 1 cup chopped tomatoes

- 1 ½ tablespoons lime juice

- 1 small onion, minced

- 2 garlic cloves, crushed

- 1 red bell pepper, deseeded and chopped

- 1 jalapeno pepper, chopped

- ¼ teaspoon oregano powder

- ½ teaspoon cumin

- ½ teaspoon coriander

- 1 tablespoon olive oil

Directions:

1. Heat the oil in a pot over medium-high flame. Add the beef to the hot oil and sear the sides until golden brown. Remove the beef from the pot and set aside.

2. Add the garlic, onions, jalapeno, oregano, cumin and coriander to the hot oil and sauté them for 2-3 minutes. Mix in the bell pepper and chopped tomatoes then stir it along with the spices. Place the beef back into the pot then season it with lime juice and Worcestershire sauce.

3. Lastly, pour in the stock then stir. Cover the pot and lower the flame to medium. Simmer the beef for 3 hours or until tender.

4. Once the beef is cooked, remove it from the pot and transfer it to a serving platter. Use a pair of forks to shred the beef into flakes. Top it with the cooked bell peppers, onions, tomatoes and some of the remaining liquid from the pot. Serve immediately.

5. This recipe makes 5 servings.

Nutrition: 233 calories; 5g sugar; 2g saturated fat; 36g protein; 8g carbohydrates; 1g fiber

Smart Points: 3

Spicy Red Ground Beef Curry

Ingredients:

- 220 grams lean ground beef
- 2 teaspoons red curry paste
- 1 ½ teaspoons coconut aminos
- 1 teaspoon minced ginger
- 1 garlic clove, crushed
- ¾ cup tomato sauce
- ½ cup coconut milk
- ½ teaspoon lemon zest
- 1 teaspoon lemon juice
- 1 leek, chopped
- 1 teaspoon olive oil

Directions:

1. Heat the olive oil in a skillet over medium-high flame. Add in the garlic, ginger and leeks and sauté them for 3 minutes. Add the beef to the skillet and let it cook for 10 minutes.

2. After 10 minutes, add the curry paste to the beef mixture and stir while cooking for 1-2 minutes. Pour in the tomato sauce, coconut aminos and lemon zest then stir. Cover the skillet and lower the flame to medium. Simmer the dish for 10 minutes.

3. Pour the lemon juice and coconut milk into the pan and stir. Continue cooking the curry for 2-3 minutes or until it has slightly thickened. Turn off the heat then transfer the curry into individual dinner plates. Serve immediately.

4. This recipe makes 2 servings.

Nutrition: 213 calories; 5g sugar; 4g saturated fat; 26g protein; 10g carbohydrates; 2g fiber

Smart Points: 4

Grilled Mozzarella Burger with Roasted Peppers

Ingredients:

- 700 grams lean ground beef

- 1 yellow bell pepper, deseeded and quartered

- 1 red bell pepper, deseeded and quartered

- 1 large onion, peeled and sliced into rings

- 2 tablespoons olive oil

- ½ teaspoon black pepper

- ¾ teaspoon paprika

- ½ teaspoon salt

- ½ teaspoon coriander

- 1 teaspoon cumin

- 1 cup shredded mozzarella cheese

Directions:

1. Heat half of the oil in a grill pan over high flame. Place the bell peppers

and onion rings on the pan and let it cook for 6-8 minutes. Once the onions have browned and the peppers have charred, remove them from the pan and let them cool on a chopping board. Gently remove the skins from the bell peppers and roughly chop the meat. Set aside.

2. In a mixing bowl, combine the ground beef, cumin, coriander, salt and paprika. Form the mixture into 6 burger patties.

3. Heat the remaining oil in the same grill pan but adjust the flame to medium-high. Place the burger patties on the pan and grill it for 5 minutes. Flip the burger over then grill it for 4 minutes.

4. In the last minute of grilling, spoon equal portions of the peppers, onions and mozzarella cheese on top of the burgers. Transfer the burgers on a serving plate. Serve with some lettuce leaves for a grain-free and low-calorie burger.

5. This recipe makes 6 servings.

Nutrition: 219 calories; 5g sugar; 4g saturated fat; 28g protein; 9g carbohydrates; 2g fiber

Smart Points: 4

Roasted Thyme and Garlic Pork Chops

Ingredients:

- 3 medium pork chops, fat trimmed off

- 2 teaspoons chopped fresh thyme

- 2 garlic cloves, minced

- Pinch of salt and black pepper

Directions:

1. Preheat the oven to 400°F.

2. Place the pork chops on a lightly-greased skillet and season the meat with thyme, garlic, salt and pepper. Let it stand for 5 minutes then place the skillet over medium-high flame. Sear each side of the pork for 3 minutes.

3. Once the pork is lightly golden in color, place the skillet in the oven and bake the chops for 8-10 minutes. Poke the meat with a fork to check for tenderness.

4. Serve the pork chops while hot.

5. This recipe makes 3 servings.

Nutrition: 195 calories; 0g sugar; 2g saturated fat; 34g protein; 1g carbohydrates; 0g fiber

Smart Points: 5

Shredded Pork and Cabbage Plate

Ingredients:

- 680 grams pork tenderloin

- 3 garlic cloves, crushed

- 4 tablespoons chicken stock

- 2 teaspoons salt

- 1 teaspoon chipotle powder

- 2 ½ cups shredded cabbage

Directions:

1. Place the pork tenderloin inside the crock pot then season it with salt, garlic and chipotle. Pour in the stock then cover it. Cook the pork on high for 3-4 hours.

2. One the last hour of cooking, add the cabbage into the crock pot. Turn off the pot then shred the meat with two forks. Stir the pork and cabbage together then transfer the dish to individual dinner plates.

3. This recipe makes 5 servings.

Nutrition: 163 calories; 1g sugar; 1g saturated fat; 30g protein; 2g carbohydrates; 1g fiber

Smart Points: 2

Oven-Baked Quinoa and Beef Meatballs

Ingredients:

- ¾ cup cooked quinoa

- 450 grams lean ground beef

- 1 egg, whisked

- 3 tablespoons grated carrots

- 2 garlic cloves, minced

- 3 tablespoons grated zucchini

- 1 small red onion, peeled and minced

- 2 tablespoons tomato sauce

- 1 tablespoon soy sauce

- ½ teaspoon oregano

- ½ teaspoon black pepper

- ½ teaspoon garlic powder

- Pinch of sea salt

Directions:

1. Preheat the oven to 425°F and prepare a parchment-lined baking sheet.

2. In a large mixing bowl, combine the beef, quinoa, carrots, zucchini, garlic, onions and tomato sauce. Mix well. Season the mixture with salt, pepper, oregano and garlic powder.

3. Knead the mixture with your hands then form 16 meatballs. Arrange the meatballs on the baking sheet then place them in the hot oven. Bake for 15 minutes or until golden brown.

4. Transfer the meatballs to smaller plates and serve hot.

5. This recipe makes 4 servings (4 meatballs per serving).

Nutrition: 150 calories; 2g sugar; 2g saturated fat; 17g protein; 8g carbohydrates; 1g fiber

Smart Points: 4

Asian-style Pork and Rice Stir-Fry

Ingredients:

- 300 grams lean ground pork
- 2 cups cooked white rice
- 2 eggs, whisked
- 2 teaspoons olive oil
- 4 garlic cloves, minced
- 2 tablespoons low-sodium soy sauce
- 1 tablespoon minced ginger
- ½ onion, peeled and minced
- 4 green onions, chopped
- 1 cup shredded cabbage
- 1 cup diced carrots
- Pinch of salt and black pepper

Directions:

1. Heat a teaspoon of oil in a pan over medium-high flame. Pour the eggs and cook them for 2 minutes. Season the egg with salt and pepper then remove it from the pan.

2. Place the ground pork into the same pan. Cook the pork for 8-10 minutes or until it turns light brown in color. Remove the pork from the pan and set aside.

3. Pour the remaining oil into the pan. Once the oil is hot, add in the garlic and onions and sauté them for 2 minutes. Mix in the carrots, cabbage, green onions and ginger and stir-fry for 2 more minutes.

4. Add the cooked white rice into the pan of vegetables and stir-fry the ingredients for 5 minutes. Finally, mix in the pork and soy sauce. Continue cooking while stirring for 3 minutes then turn off the flame.

5. Transfer the pork fried rice to smaller bowls and serve immediately.

6. This recipe makes 4 servings.

Nutrition: 386 calories; 2g sugar; 2g saturated fat; 32g protein; 44g carbohydrates; 4g fiber

Smart Points: 8

Spicy Beef and Egg Noodle Casserole

Ingredients:

- 450 grams lean ground beef

- 3 cups cooked egg noodles

- 1 cup canned cream of corn

- 1 ¾ cups tomato sauce

- 1 cup chopped red bell pepper

- 1 small onion, peeled and minced

- 3 garlic cloves, minced

- 1 cup frozen peas

- 1 tablespoon chili powder

- 1 tablespoon olive oil

- Pinch of salt

Directions:

1. Preheat the oven to 350°F and prepare a lightly-greased 3 quart baking dish.

2. Heat the oil in a pan over high flame. Add in the garlic, onions, bell peppers and beef. Cook the ingredients for 8 minutes then turn off the flame.

3. Add the egg noodles, cream of corn, tomato sauce and frozen peas into the beef mixture and mix well. Season it with salt and chili powder. Transfer the casserole mixture into the baking dish then cover the top with tin foil.

4. Bake the dish in the oven for 30-40 minutes. Serve while hot.

5. This recipe makes 6 servings.

Nutrition: 234 calories; 8g sugar; 1g saturated fat; 22g protein; 28g carbohydrates; 5g fiber

Smart Points: 6

Pan-Grilled Pineapple Pork Chops

Ingredients:

- 4 medium boneless pork chops, fat trimmed off

- 4 canned pineapple rings

- 1/3 cup pineapple juice

- 2 teaspoons corn starch

- 2 teaspoons water

- 2 tablespoons soy sauce

- 1 tablespoon brown sugar

- 1 table spoon apple cider vinegar

- ½ teaspoon garlic powder

- ½ teaspoon minced fresh ginger

- ½ teaspoon ground black pepper

- 1 tablespoon olive oil

Directions:

1. Dissolve the corn starch in water and set aside. In a separate bowl, mix together the pineapple juice, brown

sugar, vinegar, soy sauce, garlic powder, black pepper and ginger.

2. Place the pork chops in a large Ziploc bag then pour in the pineapple soy mixture. Seal the bag them place it in the fridge. Marinate the pork chops overnight.

3. The following day, take out the pork chops from the fridge then remove it from the marinade. Let it drain on a colander.

4. Place the marinade in a saucepan over medium flame. Mix in the corn starch slurry then simmer the sauce for 2 minutes or until it begins to thicken. Remove the saucepan from the flame then set aside.

5. Preheat the grill pan on the stovetop. Grease the pan with the olive oil then place the pineapple slices on it. Grill each side for 2 minutes then set aside.

6. Once the pineapples have been grilled, arrange the pork chops on the pan then grill each side for 5

minutes. Use a bit of the pineapple soy sauce to baste the meat.

7. Transfer the pork chops to smaller plates then top it with a pineapple ring. Drizzle the sauce over the dish then serve immediately.

8. This recipe makes 4 servings.

Nutrition: 200 calories; 8g sugar; 2g saturated fat; 25g protein; 9g carbohydrates; 1g fiber

Smart Points: 5

Chapter 7 Fish and Seafood Recipes

Sautéed Lemon and Herb Shrimp

Ingredients:

- 450 grams large shrimp, peeled and deveined

- 1 teaspoon lemon pepper seasoning

- 2 tablespoons lemon juice

- 2 tablespoons chopped parsley

- 2 teaspoons olive oil

- Pinch of salt and black pepper

Directions:

1. Heat the oil in a skillet over medium-high flame. Once the oil is hot, add the shrimps and sauté for 1 minute.

2. After 1 minute, add in the lemon juice, lemon pepper seasoning, salt and pepper. Continue cooking the shrimp for 3 minutes or until the shrimp has turned pink.

3. Turn off the flame then add in the parsley. Toss the dish then serve immediately.

4. This recipe makes 4 servings.

Nutrition: 103 calories; 0g sugar; 0g saturated fat; 16g protein; 2g carbohydrates; 0g fiber

Smart Points: 3

Grilled Halibut with Tomato and Lima Beans

Ingredients:

- 2 halibut fillets, sliced in half

- 1 ¾ cups canned lima beans, drained

- 8 cherry tomatoes, halved

- 4 basil leaves, chopped

- 2 green onions, chopped

- 2 tablespoons olive oil

- 1 tablespoon water

- Pinch of salt and black pepper

Directions:

1. Season the halibut fillets with salt and pepper. Moisten the grill pan with cooking spray then cook the fillets over medium-high flame until both sides are golden brown. Set aside the fish.

2. Heat the oil in a pan over medium flame. Sauté the onions in the hot oil until translucent then add in the

basil and tomatoes. Continue cooking the vegetables for 3 minutes.

3. Pour in the lima beans and water then continue cooking for 2 minutes. Turn off the flame then sprinkle green onions on top of the vegetables.

4. Place the fillets on dinner plates then spoon the tomato and bean mixture on top. Serve immediately.

5. This recipe makes 4 servings.

Nutrition: 307 calories; 1g sugar; 2g saturated fat; 23g protein; 22g carbohydrates; 7g fiber

Smart Points: 8

Rosemary Salmon Skewers

Ingredients:

- 500 grams wild salmon, sliced into 12 cubes

- 3 tablespoons fresh rosemary

- 2 tablespoons olive oil

- 1 tablespoon mustard

- 2 tablespoons lemon juice

- ½ teaspoon black pepper

- ½ teaspoon garlic powder

- ½ teaspoon sea salt

- 4 wooden skewers, pre-soaked in water

Directions:

1. Place the salmon in a bowl then pour in the olive oil, mustard and lemon juice. Season the fish with salt, pepper and garlic powder then stir it gently. Let the fish marinade for 30 minutes. After 30 minutes, skewer 3

pieces of salmon into each stick and set aside.

2. Heat the griller to high then moisten the grate with cooking spray. Once the grill is hot, lay the salmon skewers on the grate and roast it for 6-8 minutes, turning every 2 minutes. Baste it with the remaining marinade.

3. Serve the salmon skewers warm.

4. This recipe makes 4 servings.

Nutrition: 308 calories; 0g sugar; 5g saturated fat; 24g protein; 2g carbohydrates; 1g fiber

SmartPoints: 8

Baked Tilapia and Parmesan Fillet

Ingredients:

- 3 medium tilapia fillets

- 4 tablespoons bread crumbs

- ½ cup grated Parmesan cheese

- 2 tablespoons olive oil

- 2 teaspoons garlic powder

- 2 teaspoons paprika

- 1 tablespoon dried parsley

Directions:

1. Preheat the oven to 400°F and prepare a parchment-lined baking sheet.

2. Combine the bread crumbs, Parmesan cheese, paprika, garlic powder and dried parsley in a large bowl. Place the tilapia fillets in the bowl then rub the breading all over the fish.

3. Arrange the breaded tilapia on the baking sheet then drizzle olive oil on

top of it. Bake the fish for 15-20 minutes or until golden brown.

4. Transfer the fillets to individual dinner plates and serve immediately.

5. This recipe makes 3 servings.

Nutrition: 189 calories; 0g sugar; 3g saturated fat; 24g protein; 2g carbohydrates; 1g fiber

SmartPoints: 4

Lime and Garlic Shrimp Kabobs

Ingredients:

- 18 pieces large shrimp, peeled and deveined

- ½ cup lime juice

- 4 garlic cloves, minced

- 2 tablespoons olive oil

- ¼ teaspoon paprika

- ¼ teaspoon lemon pepper seasoning

- 2 tablespoons chopped parsley

- 6 metal skewers

Directions:

1. Combine olive oil, garlic, lime juice, paprika, lemon pepper seasoning and raw shrimp. Place the marinated shrimp in the fridge for 15 minutes. After 15 minutes, take out the shrimps from the fridge then skewer 3 shrimps into each stick. Set aside.

2. Heat a grill pan over medium-high flame. Place the shrimp skewers on

the pan and grill them for 4-5 minutes, using the remaining marinade to baste the seafood. Once the shrimps turn bright pink, serve it immediately.

3. This recipe makes 6 servings.

Nutrition: 108 calories; 0g sugar; 1g saturated fat; 15g protein; 1g carbohydrates; 0g fiber

Smart Points: 2

Whole Wheat Shrimp Salad Burrito

Ingredients:

- 170 grams cooked shrimp, minced
- 4 tablespoons canned black-eyed peas, drained
- 4 tablespoons canned corn kernels, drained
- 1 cup shredded lettuce
- 4 tablespoons chopped fresh cilantro
- 6 tablespoons salsa
- 1 teaspoon chili powder
- ¼ teaspoon cumin
- 4 tablespoons sour cream
- 1 tablespoon lime juice
- 2 whole wheat tortillas
- 1 teaspoon salt

Directions:

1. Combine the shrimp, black-eyed peas, corn, lettuce, cilantro, salsa and sour cream. Season the burrito filling with chili powder, cumin and salt. Toss the mixture gently.

2. Heat the tortillas on a pan over medium flame then place each of them on a plate. Spoon equal portions of the shrimp filling at the middle of the tortilla then fold both sides towards the center. Secure the burrito by wrapping it in wax paper. Serve immediately.

3. This recipe makes 2 servings.

Nutrition: 277 calories; 6.5 g sugar; 1g saturated fat; 27g protein; 40g carbohydrates; 8g fiber

SmartPoints: 6

Braised Cod with Tomato and Thyme Sauce

Ingredients:

- 4 cod fillets

- 1 ¾ cups chopped tomatoes

- ½ cup minced onions

- 3 teaspoons fresh thyme

- 2 garlic cloves, minced

- ¼ cup heavy cream

- ¾ cup white wine

- ½ teaspoon corn starch

- ½ teaspoon salt

- ¼ teaspoon ground black pepper

- 1 tablespoon olive oil

Directions:

1. Place the cod fillets on a plate then season it with half of the salt, a teaspoon of thyme and black pepper. Set aside.

2. Heat the olive oil in a pan over medium flame. Add the garlic and onions and sauté for one minute. Once the onions are translucent, add in the cod, tomatoes and wine then cover the pan. Let the dish simmer for 5 minutes. Once the fish is cooked, gently remove it from the pan then place it on a serving bowl. Set aside.

3. Pour the corn starch and cream into the pan with the tomatoes and wine. Sprinkle the remaining salt and thyme into the sauce and stir continuously while cooking. Once the sauce starts to thicken, turn off the flame.

4. Using a spoon, pour the tomato sauce over the cod. Serve immediately.

5. This recipe makes 4 servings.

Nutrition: 227 calories; 0g sugar; 4g saturated fat; 19g protein; 7g carbohydrates; 1g fiber

SmartPoints: 6

Seared Scallops with Sweet Mustard Sauce

Ingredients:

- 450 grams sea scallops, patted dry
- 1 tablespoon mustard
- 1 ½ tablespoons honey
- ½ tablespoon cane vinegar
- 1 ½ tablespoons soy sauce
- ¼ teaspoon red pepper flakes
- 1 teaspoon toasted sesame seeds
- 1 tablespoon olive oil

Directions:

1. Whisk together mustard, honey, cane vinegar, soy sauce and pepper flakes. Set aside.

2. Heat the oil in a pan over medium-high flame. Place the scallops in the hot oil and cook for 2 minutes. Flip the scallops over and cook for

another 2 minutes. Transfer the scallops to a plate and set aside.

3. Pour the mustard sauce into the same pan, adjust the heat to medium then let it simmer until thick. Once the sauce has reduced, turn off the flame then place the scallops back into the pan. Stir until the scallops are coated with the sauce.

4. Transfer the scallops into smaller plates then sprinkle toasted sesame seeds on top. Serve immediately.

5. This recipe makes 4 servings.

Nutrition: 180 calories; 4g sugar; 1g saturated fat; 20g protein; 10g carbohydrates; 0g fiber

SmartPoints: 4

Three-Cheese Tuna Casserole

Ingredients:

- 1 ¼ cups canned tuna, flaked
- 1 cup chopped button mushrooms
- 4 cups cooked whole wheat macaroni noodles
- 1 small onion, minced
- 1 cup frozen green peas, thawed
- 1 cup grated cheddar cheese
- 1 cup milk
- 1 cup cottage cheese
- ¾ cup grated Parmesan cheese
- 2 tablespoons olive oil
- Pinch of salt and black pepper

Directions:

1. Preheat the oven to 375°F and prepare a 3-quart baking dish. Grease the dish with a tablespoon of the oil.

2. Heat the remaining oil in a pan over medium-high flame. Sauté the onions and mushrooms for 5 minutes. Add in the tuna and green peas then continue cooking for another 5 minutes. Turn off the flame.

3. Pour the tuna and mushroom mixture into a large bowl. Mix in the macaroni, milk, cheddar cheese and cottage cheese. Toss the casserole then season it with salt and pepper.

4. Transfer the mixture into the baking dish then sprinkle parmesan cheese on top. Bake the casserole in the oven for 15 minutes. Let the casserole cool for 10 minutes before serving.

5. This recipe makes 6 servings.

Nutrition: 300 calories; 5g sugar; 3g saturated fat; 31g protein; 24g carbohydrates; 5g fiber

SmartPoints: 6

Baked Flounder with Almond Crust

Ingredients:

- 200 grams flounder fillet, halved

- 3 tablespoons finely-ground almonds

- ¼ teaspoon salt

- 1 teaspoon olive oil

- ½ teaspoon black pepper

- ½ teaspoon garlic powder

Directions:

1. Preheat the oven to 350°F and prepare a parchment-lined baking sheet.

2. Place the fillets in a bowl then season it with salt and pepper. Sprinkle the ground almonds onto the fish then toss until well-coated. Press the nuts on the fish to prevent them from falling off.

3. Lay the fillets on the baking sheet, drizzle olive oil on top of it then place

them in the oven. Bake the fillets for 20 minutes.

4. Let the fish cool on a wire rack for 10 minutes then serve.

5. This recipe makes 2 servings.

Nutrition: 248 calories; 1g sugar; 3g saturated fat; 16g protein; 10g carbohydrates; 4g fiber

SmartPoints: 7

Conclusion

Thank you again for buying this book!

I hope this book was able to convince you to try out Weight Watchers' SmartPoints system as a means to lose weight the healthy way. It is a revolutionary weight loss system that allows you to easily calculate food points with the objective of achieving a healthier body, mind and spirit. You must realize that mindful eating really does make you look good and feel good about yourself.

In addition to that, the recipes in this book are made from healthy and clean ingredients that are low in SmartPoints. This means that if you are planning to lose a significant amount of body fat, then these recipes will definitely help you reach your fitness goals. What's even better about these 50 recipes is that the SmartPoints have already been listed for you, thus you no longer need to calculate nutritional values or purchase a Weight Watchers calculator. These recipes will make it very convenient for you to cook and change your eating habits for the better.

To make your weight loss journey a success, it would be beneficial for you to use this book as a guide to making positive and long-term changes in your life. May you be inspired by the story of Jean Nidetch and hopefully find that inner desire to make smarter life choices that will position you in a path towards reaching your dreams.

Made in the USA
Middletown, DE
29 September 2016